THE FACTS ABOUT DIABETES

THINGS YOU NEED TO KNOW

LIZZIE HOWE

Table of contents

Introduction

Diabetes is a chronic condition brought on by either insufficient insulin production by the pancreas or inefficient insulin utilization by the body. The insulin hormone regulates blood sugar levels. Uncontrolled diabetes frequently causes hyperglycemia, also known as high blood sugar or raised blood glucose, which over time causes substantial harm to numerous bodily systems, including the neurons and blood vessels. 8.5% of persons who were 18 years of age and older had diabetes in 2014. In 2019, 1.5 million people died as a direct result of diabetes, with people under the age of 70 accounting for 48% of these deaths. High blood glucose is to blame for 20% of cardiovascular mortality, and diabetes contributed to an additional 460 000 deaths from renal illness. In 2019, 1.5 million people died as a direct result of diabetes, with people under the age of 70 accounting for 48% of these deaths. High blood glucose is to blame for 20% of cardiovascular mortality, and diabetes contributed to an additional 460 000 deaths from renal illness.

Age-standardized diabetes mortality rates increased by 3% between 2000 and 2019.

In lower-middle-income countries, the mortality rates from diabetes increased by 13%.

On the other hand, the chance of passing away from any of the four major noncommunicable diseases (cancer, chronic respiratory diseases, diabetes, or cardiovascular diseases) between the ages of 30 and 70 decreased globally by 22% between 2000 and 2019.

Diabetes symptoms can strike unexpectedly. The modest symptoms of type 2 diabetes may not be seen for many years.
Blood arteries in the kidneys, eyes, heart, and nerves can suffer damage

from diabetes over time. Renal failure, heart attack, and stroke risk factors for diabetes are all increased.

Diabetes can cause irreversible vision loss by affecting the blood vessels in the eyes. Many persons with diabetes experience foot problems because of nerve damage and insufficient blood supply. This might cause foot sores and perhaps call for an amputation. To avoid type 2 diabetes' worst side effects, early diagnosis is crucial. The easiest method to catch diabetes early is to visit a doctor regularly for checkups and blood tests.

Type 2 diabetes can have modest symptoms. It could be years before anyone notices them.

The signs of type 2 diabetes can be similar to those of type 1, although being less severe most of the time. As a result, it's possible that the problem won't be discovered until after issues have developed.

Type 2 diabetes affects more than 95% of those who have the disease. Previously known as adult-onset or non-insulin dependent type 2 diabetes. This type of diabetes was previously exclusively found in adults, but it is now increasingly common in kids as well.

Hyperglycemia during pregnancy occurs when blood glucose levels are above normal but below those that are indicative of diabetes.

When a woman becomes pregnant, gestational diabetes may manifest. Women with gestational diabetes have a higher risk of pregnancy and delivery complications. These women are more likely to develop type 2 diabetes later in life, as are perhaps their offspring. Prenatal screening is used to determine gestational diabetes rather than patient reports of symptoms.

Chapter 1

Diabetes definition

Diabetes is a long-term medical illness that interferes with your body's ability to control blood sugar (glucose). Your body uses glucose, which is obtained from food, as a major source of energy. The pancreas secretes the hormone insulin, which aids in transporting glucose from the bloodstream to your cells, where it can be used as fuel.

Diabetes patients have problems with either insulin production or insulin metabolism. Hyperglycemia, or increased blood glucose levels, are the result of this. The three primary kinds of diabetes are as follows:

Type 1 diabetes is an autoimmune condition in which the immune system unintentionally targets and kills the pancreatic cells that make insulin. The body thus produces little to no insulin. People with type 1 diabetes must use an insulin pump or administer insulin injections to control their blood sugar levels. Diabetes type 1 typically first appears in childhood or adolescence.

The most prevalent type of diabetes, type 2, typically develops in maturity but can happen at any age. In type 2 diabetes, the body either stops producing enough insulin to meet the body's demands or develops a resistance to the effects of insulin. Obesity, a sedentary lifestyle, a family history of the disease, and certain ethnic backgrounds are all type 2 diabetes risk factors. Changes in lifestyle, such as a nutritious diet, regular exercise, and occasionally oral medicines or insulin, can frequently control type 2 diabetes.

Diabetes of this type, known as gestational diabetes, normally goes away after the baby is born. Hormonal changes that interfere with insulin function are the cause of it, which affects roughly 2–10% of pregnant women. Blood sugar levels must be closely monitored for gestational diabetes, which may also necessitate dietary adjustments, physical activity, or insulin therapy.

Diabetes can cause several complications, such as heart disease, stroke, kidney disease, nerve damage, and eye issues if it is not properly managed.

However, people with diabetes can live active, satisfying lives if they receive the right medical attention, regularly check their blood sugar levels, and adopt a healthy lifestyle. It's crucial to collaborate closely with healthcare specialists to create a customized management plan that meets your unique requirements.

Chapter 2

Diabetes Causes & Risk Factors

Diabetes Causes

When the body is unable to control blood glucose levels, diabetes, a chronic medical condition, develops. Type 1 diabetes and type 2 diabetes are the two basic kinds of the disease. The root causes and risk factors for each category are listed below:

Diabetes Type 1:

1. Autoimmune Response: In type 1 diabetes, the immune system unintentionally targets and kills the pancreatic cells that make insulin. Even though the precise aetiology of this autoimmune reaction is not entirely understood, genetic and environmental factors are thought to be involved.

2. Genetic Propensity: Type 1 diabetes is more likely to develop in those who carry specific genes.

However, the presence of these genes does not ensure the onset of the illness, indicating that additional variables may be at play.

3. Environmental Triggers: In people who are genetically predisposed to type 1 diabetes, certain environmental events, such as virus infections or exposure to specific chemicals, may set off the autoimmune response.

Diabetes Type 2:

1. Insulin Resistance: Type 2 diabetes develops when the body either stops producing enough insulin to meet its demands or becomes resistant to the effects of insulin. Controlling blood sugar levels is made possible by the hormone insulin. The body's cells could eventually develop insulin resistance, which would result in high blood sugar levels.

2. Obesity and Sedentary Lifestyle: Type 2 diabetes is significantly more likely to occur in those who are overweight or obese. Insulin resistance is exacerbated by excess body fat, particularly in the abdominal region. Insulin resistance can also occur as a result of inactivity and a sedentary lifestyle.

3. Genetics and Family History: Both genetics and family history have an impact on type 2 diabetes.
Your chance of getting type 2 diabetes is increased if you have close relatives who have the disease.

4. Age and Ethnicity: Type 2 diabetes risk rises with age, particularly after age 45. African-Americans, Hispanic/Latino

Americans, Native Americans, and Asian Americans all have a higher risk of developing type 2 diabetes than other ethnic groups.

5. Gestational Diabetes: Type 2 diabetes in later life is more likely to strike women who have experienced gestational diabetes during pregnancy.

It's crucial to remember that although these factors raise a person's risk of getting diabetes, they do not guarantee that they will. Other uncommon types of diabetes exist as well, including gestational diabetes, which develops during pregnancy and is impacted by hormonal changes.

Diabetes Risk Factors

Numerous risk factors can raise a person's chance of developing diabetes. The kind of diabetes can affect these risk factors differently. The following are typical risk factors for both type 1 and type 2 diabetes:

Diabetes Type 1 Risk Factors:

1. Family History: Having a close relative with type 1 diabetes, such as a parent or sibling, increases the risk of getting the disease.

2. Genetic Predisposition: Some genes are linked to a higher risk of developing type 1 diabetes.
However, the presence of these genes does not ensure the disease will manifest.

3. Age: Type 1 diabetes can manifest at any age, but it's most frequently discovered in kids, teenagers, and young adults.

Diabetes Type 2 Risk Factors:

1. Obesity or Overweight: A major risk factor for type 2 diabetes is being overweight or obese. Insulin resistance is exacerbated by excess body fat, especially around the abdomen (central obesity).

2. Sedentary Lifestyle: Lack of exercise and a sedentary lifestyle both raise the risk of type 2 diabetes and the development of insulin resistance.

3. Family History: Type 2 diabetes doubles the likelihood of getting the disease if a parent or sibling has it.

4. Age: As people get older, especially after the age of 45, their risk of type 2 diabetes rises.

5. Ethnicity: Type 2 diabetes is more common in some ethnic groups, including African-Americans, Hispanic/Latino Americans, Native Americans, Asian Americans, and Pacific Islanders.

6. Gestational Diabetes: Type 2 diabetes in later life is more likely to strike women who have experienced gestational diabetes during pregnancy.

7. Hypertension: Having high blood pressure (also known as hypertension) is linked to a higher risk of type 2 diabetes.

8. Abnormal Cholesterol Levels: Type 2 diabetes risk can be increased by abnormally low levels of HDL (good) cholesterol and/or excessive levels of triglycerides.

9. Polycystic Ovary Syndrome (PCOS): Type 2 diabetes is more likely to develop in women with PCOS, a hormonal condition marked by irregular periods and high levels of androgen.

10. Sleep Disorders: Type 2 diabetes risk is exacerbated by conditions including obstructive sleep apnea.

It's crucial to remember that a person's risk for developing diabetes is not always determined by the presence of these risk factors.

However, they show a higher chance of getting the ailment, so people with these risk factors must take preventive actions, such as leading a healthy lifestyle and getting frequent medical checkups.

Chapter 3

Diabetes Symptoms

Depending on the kind of diabetes and the person, the symptoms of diabetes might change. The following are some typical signs and symptoms of diabetes:

1. Frequent Urination (Polyuria):
One of the initial symptoms of diabetes is frequent urination. Increased urination occurs when blood sugar levels are high because the kidneys try to flush the extra glucose from the body through urine.

2. Excessive Thirst (Polydipsia):
Dehydration brought on by increased urination might result in excessive thirst. Diabetes patients frequently feel they need to hydrate themselves more than usual.

3. Unexplained Weight Loss: Type 1 diabetes causes the body to start metabolizing fat and muscle for energy because it lacks insulin, making it difficult for the body to utilize glucose properly. This causes weight loss despite adequate dietary intake. Weight loss may occur in people with type 2 diabetes because their bodies may not generate or utilize insulin as effectively as they should.

4. Increased Hunger (Polyphagia): People with diabetes may experience prolonged hunger despite eating more than normal. This happens as a result of the body's cells not getting enough glucose for energy.

5. Fatigue and Weakness: People with diabetes may experience fatigue, weakness, and a lack of energy as a result of their body's inability to utilize glucose properly. Reduced energy levels are caused by inadequate insulin or insulin resistance, which blocks glucose from entering the cells.

6. Blurred Vision: High blood sugar levels can result in the removal of fluid from the eye lenses, which can cause blurred vision. As soon as blood sugar levels are under control, this symptom can become better.

7. Slow Healing of Wounds: Diabetes can impair a person's body's capacity for normal healing. It could take longer for cuts, wounds, and infections to heal.

8. Tingling or Numbness: Long-term blood sugar elevations can harm nerves, resulting in diabetic neuropathy. This might result in burning, tingling, or numbness, usually in the hands, feet, or legs.

9. Recurring Infections: Diabetes can impair immune function, leaving people more prone to infections. Urinary tract infections, yeast infections, and skin infections are examples of typical infections.

It's significant to remember that these symptoms might potentially be related to other illnesses. It is advised that you speak with a healthcare expert for an accurate examination and diagnosis if you encounter any of these symptoms.

Chapter 4

Diabetes's Effects

High blood sugar levels are a symptom of diabetes, a chronic medical disorder caused by either an inability of the body to make insulin (Type 1 diabetes) or an inefficient utilization of insulin (Type 2 diabetes).

Diabetes can have a wide range of negative impacts on the body's systems and organs. Here are a few typical diabetic effects:

1. Cardiovascular issues: Diabetic patients are much more likely to experience cardiovascular complications like peripheral artery disease, heart attacks, and strokes. Blood vessels can be harmed by elevated blood sugar levels, which increases the risk of cardiovascular issues and causes atherosclerosis (the hardening and constriction of arteries).

2. Nerve damage (neuropathy): People with diabetes are more likely to experience nerve damage in their legs and feet than in other parts of the body. This may result in symptoms like tingling, discomfort, numbness, and loss of sensation. In extreme circumstances, it may also impair sexual, urinary, and digestive functions.

3. Nephropathy, or damage to the kidneys: Diabetes is one of the main factors contributing to kidney failure. Long-term high blood sugar levels can harm the kidneys' small blood capillaries, making it harder for them to remove waste and extra fluid from the blood.
Toxin buildup and chronic kidney disease development may arise from this.

4. Eye issues (retinopathy): Diabetes can harm the blood vessels in the retina, the tissue at the back of the eye that is sensitive to light. Diabetic retinopathy is a disorder that, if untreated, can cause vision issues and ultimately blindness.

5. Enhanced risk of infections: People with diabetes are more prone to several diseases, including skin, fungus, and urinary tract infections.

High blood sugar levels foster the growth of microorganisms and make the immune system less effective at warding off diseases.

6. The body's normal healing mechanism may be hampered by diabetes. Blood circulation and the immune system are impacted by high blood sugar levels, which makes it harder for wounds to heal. This might result in persistent wounds that don't heal, especially in the lower extremities, which raises the danger of infection and other problems.

7. Enhanced risk of additional complications: Diabetes is linked to an increased risk of some additional health issues, such as high blood pressure, high cholesterol, obesity, sleep apnea, and some types of cancer. It may also be detrimental to mental health, raising the chance of cognitive decline, sadness, and anxiety.

Effective diabetes care includes taking medicine, making lifestyle changes (such as eating a nutritious diet, exercising frequently, and managing weight), and routinely checking blood sugar levels.

Diabetes should be managed properly to lower the likelihood and severity of these consequences. To properly manage diabetes and lessen its long-term effects, it is essential to seek the advice of healthcare specialists and adhere to their recommendations.

Chapter 5

Treatment and diagnosis

Symptoms, medical history, and different tests are commonly used to diagnose diabetes. Type 1 diabetes, type 2 diabetes, and gestational diabetes are the three most prevalent kinds of the disease.

1. Type 1 diabetes: Children and young people are typically diagnosed with this kind.

It happens when the body's immune system unintentionally targets and kills the pancreatic cells that make insulin. Frequent urination, excessive thirst, unexplained weight loss, intense hunger, weariness, and blurred vision are all possible signs of type 1 diabetes.

2. Type 2 diabetes: This form is more prevalent and is frequently linked to lifestyle choices like weight and inactivity. To maintain normal blood sugar levels, the body must either create adequate insulin or develop resistance to the effects of insulin.

Frequent urination, increased thirst, unexplained weight loss or gain, weariness, hazy vision, slowly healing wounds, and recurrent infections are all signs of type 2 diabetes.

3. Gestational diabetes: This form of diabetes normally disappears after childbirth and develops throughout pregnancy. It is identified during normal prenatal screening exams to check blood sugar levels.

The following tests may be used by medical experts to identify diabetes:

1. The fasting plasma glucose (FPG) test analyzes your blood sugar level after a minimum of eight hours of fasting. Diabetes is often identified by readings of 126 mg/dL or greater on two different occasions.

2. Oral glucose tolerance test (OGTT): You sip a sweet beverage after having your blood sugar tested after a fast. Over the subsequent few hours, blood sugar levels are checked at regular intervals. After two hours, a blood sugar level of 200 mg/dL or greater may signify diabetes.

3. Your average blood sugar levels over the previous two to three months are measured by the hemoglobin A1c (HbA1c) test. Diabetes is often indicated by an HbA1c reading of 6.5% or greater on two distinct occasions.

These tests aid medical practitioners in the diagnosis of diabetes and the selection of the right type and course of therapy. It's crucial to speak with a healthcare professional for a precise diagnosis and tailored advice based on your unique circumstances.

Treatment

Diabetes is normally treated with a mix of medicine, lifestyle changes, and, occasionally, insulin therapy. The specific course of therapy is determined by the type of diabetes and personal characteristics. An overview of diabetic treatment options is provided below:

Type 1 Diabetes: Since type 1 diabetics' bodies are unable to manufacture insulin, they need insulin therapy. An insulin pump or several daily injections might be used to deliver the insulin.

Other crucial components of managing type 1 diabetes are regular physical activity, carbohydrate counting, and blood sugar monitoring.

Type 2 Diabetes: Treatment for type 2 diabetes focuses on lifestyle modifications, including adopting a nutritious diet, increasing physical exercise, decreasing weight where necessary, and monitoring blood sugar levels. Additionally, prescription drugs may be given to assist control blood sugar levels. These can consist of oral drugs that boost insulin production, improve insulin sensitivity, or lessen hepatic glucose production.

In some situations, insulin therapy might be required if other methods of blood sugar control are insufficient.

Gestational Diabetes: Through diet and exercise, pregnant women with gestational diabetes may be able to manage their blood sugar levels. However, some women might need to take insulin or oral drugs throughout pregnancy to manage their condition.

In addition to these methods of treatment, several broader strategies can aid in managing diabetes:

Blood Sugar Monitoring: It's crucial to regularly check your blood sugar levels to adapt your treatment and keep everything under control.

Healthy Diet: Blood sugar levels can be regulated by eating a balanced diet that contains a range of fruits, vegetables, whole grains, lean meats, and healthy fats. Limiting the consumption of sweetened meals and beverages is crucial.

Regular Physical Activity: Regular physical activity can help lower blood sugar levels and enhance general health.

Adherence to Medication: To effectively control diabetes, it is essential to take prescription medications when prescribed and in specified amounts.

Routine Checkups: Monitoring blood sugar levels, making necessary treatment plan modifications, and controlling any consequences all depend on regular checkups with medical specialists.

Diabetes care is extremely customized, and treatment strategies may change depending on a person's particular requirements and circumstances.

Determining the best course of treatment for a diabetic patient requires consultation with a healthcare provider or a diabetes care team.

Chapter 6

Why Does Diabetes Affect Wound Healing?

When you have diabetes, your body behaves somewhat differently from when you don't.

If you have diabetes, your body either cannot naturally generate insulin or cannot use it efficiently. You can end up needing frequent blood sugar checks and artificial insulin as a result of this. It also implies that injuries could not heal as quickly or effectively as they would in a body free of diabetes.

Understanding how diabetes can impact wound healing and being aware of the significance of good wound care and management are imperative if you or someone you love has the disease.

Untreated diabetic wounds can soon get infected, which can lead to major problems like the need for surgery, foot ulcers, or even amputation.

Chapter 7

The Impact of Diabetes on Proper Wound Healing

1. Chronic Inflammation Is a Common Complication in Diabetics

Wounds become inflamed during the second stage of healing. Diabetic wounds can take too long to heal at this stage, turning them into "chronic" wounds. If a wound persists for six months or more, it is deemed chronic.

2. Increased Levels of Blood Sugar

One of the most crucial things that diabetics need to think about is keeping a good blood sugar level because diabetes restricts how the body can handle glucose. How quickly your wounds heal is greatly influenced by your blood sugar levels.

For instance, when these levels are excessively high in diabetics, the immune system's ability to operate, the ability of nutrients and oxygen to energize cells, and inflammation levels all rise. All of which may prevent wounds from healing effectively.

3. Diabetic Neuropathy

In addition to making the arteries rigid, high blood sugar can also induce diabetic neuropathy and narrow blood vessels. Damaged nerves all over the body lead to diabetic neuropathy. It results in tingling and numbness in the limbs, making it challenging to feel your injuries.

This may result in fresh wounds and difficulties with general recovery.

Because of this, it's crucial for diabetics to frequently check their skin, particularly the bottoms of their feet.

4. Issues with Circulation

When the body's blood is properly circulated, wounds heal significantly more quickly. Due to their restricted blood vessels, diabetics often have impaired circulation and are more susceptible to developing illnesses like peripheral vascular disease.

Diabetes patients may have lower oxygen levels, which can slow down tissue growth and, in turn, wound healing.

5. Ineffective Immune System Response

High blood sugar levels impair the function of red and white blood cells, which lowers the amount of nutrients that can be delivered to the wound site to fight infections. This is also brought on by the fact that a diabetic body produces specific hormones that weaken the immune system.

Your body may have a harder time fighting off bacteria if your immune system isn't working properly, which can hinder wound healing and increase your risk of infection.

6. Enhanced Infection Risk

White blood cell mobility is slower in diabetic individuals than in healthy people. This indicates that the immune system is not working as well, which causes wounds to become more inflammatory. The wound may deteriorate as a result of this in addition to neuropathy-related numbness.

As previously mentioned, there is a higher risk of infection when an open incision heals more slowly than it would otherwise. Increased rates of gangrene, sepsis, and infections like osteomyelitis are frequently the result of this. The leading cause of amputations of all limbs each year is diabetic ulcers.

Chapter 8

Renal and eye effects of diabetes

Impacts on the kidney

Diabetes, which is one of the main causes of diabetic nephropathy, can have a substantial negative impact on the kidneys. Following are some renal effects of diabetes:

1. Elevated blood sugar levels: Diabetes-related high blood sugar levels can harm the body's blood vessels, especially the tiny blood vessels in the kidneys. Kidney function may eventually be compromised as a result of this.

2. Glomerular damage: The glomeruli, which are microscopic filters found in the kidneys that assist in removing waste and surplus fluid from the circulation, are damaged.

Glomerulosclerosis, a condition brought on by damaged glomeruli, is a result of elevated blood sugar levels. Toxins may build up in the body as a result of the kidney's inability to filter waste products efficiently.

3. Elevated blood pressure: Another risk factor for kidney disease, diabetes can also increase blood pressure (also known as hypertension). The kidneys' capacity to work properly can be hampered by high blood pressure, which can further damage the blood vessels there.

4. Albuminuria: Albuminuria, or the presence of extra protein (albumin) in the urine, is one of the early symptoms of diabetic nephropathy. When the kidneys are healthy, protein does not leak through the damaged filters into the urine, but when they are damaged, protein can.
Albuminuria that persists over time is a sign of renal damage and can lead to more advanced kidney disease.

5. Reduced kidney function: As diabetes worsens, the kidneys' capacity to filter waste materials and control fluid balance decreases. This can culminate in chronic kidney disease (CKD), a disorder marked by a reduction in kidney function. To maintain their health, those with severe CKD may need dialysis or a kidney transplant. To lower the risk of renal issues, it's crucial for diabetics to carefully monitor and control their blood sugar levels, blood pressure, and kidney function.

The effects of diabetes on the kidneys can be lessened by regular medical checkups, adherence to recommended medications, and lifestyle changes like eating healthily and exercising.

Diabetes's Effects on the Eye

Diabetes can significantly affect the eyes and cause many issues that are related to the eyes. Diabetic retinopathy is the most typical eye problem brought on by diabetes. Here are some effects of diabetes on the eyes:

1. Diabetic Retinopathy: The blood vessels in the retina, the light-sensitive tissue at the back of the eye, can be harmed by high blood sugar levels over an extended period. Adult blindness is most commonly caused by diabetic retinopathy. Blood vessels may bleed or leak fluid as a result, causing retinal oedema and vision issues.

2. Diabetic Macular Edema (DME): DME is a specific type of diabetic

retinopathy in which fluid leaking causes the macula, the area in the centre of the retina that is responsible for clear, central vision, to swell.
If neglected, this illness can result in hazy or distorted vision as well as serious vision loss.

3. Cataracts: Diabetics are more likely to experience cataract development. Vision blur is caused by a cataract, which is the clouding of the eye's natural lens. Cataract development and advancement may be sped up by diabetes.

4. Glaucoma: A series of eye diseases known as glaucoma that harm the optic nerve are more likely to occur in people with diabetes. Increased intraocular pressure damages the optic nerve and impairs vision.

Neovascular glaucoma is a specific type of glaucoma that may be more common in people with diabetes.

5. Dry Eyes: Diabetes can result in dry eyes, which are characterized by insufficient tear production to maintain comfortable and moisturized eyes. This may cause gritty sensations, ocular discomfort, and an elevated risk of eye infections.

To monitor and identify any early eye-related issues, people with diabetes must get routine eye exams by an eye care specialist.

Adopting a healthy lifestyle and managing blood pressure, cholesterol, blood sugar, and blood sugar levels will help lower the risk and advancement of certain eye conditions.

Chapter 9

Diabetes and Hypertension

Does diabetes have any effect on blood pressure? Diabetes can help high blood pressure develop. Oftentimes, diabetes and high blood pressure coexist; this condition is referred to as "diabetic hypertension." The following factors could be a link between the two ailments:

1. Insulin resistance: Type 2 diabetes is characterized by the body's development of immunity to the effects of insulin, which raises blood sugar levels. Additionally, blood arteries may be affected by insulin resistance, tightening and increasing blood pressure.

2. Kidney function: Over time, diabetes can harm the kidneys, causing a condition known as diabetic nephropathy.

Blood pressure may rise when the kidneys are damaged because they may be unable to remove waste and extra fluid from the body as efficiently.

3. Chronic inflammation and endothelial dysfunction: Diabetes is linked to endothelial dysfunction or faulty blood vessel lining function. These elements may hinder the blood vessels' capacity to dilate and relax, which heightens blood pressure.

4. Obesity: Type 2 diabetes and obesity are frequently linked, and obesity also increases the risk of high blood pressure.
Inflammation, insulin resistance, and other metabolic problems brought on by excess weight might increase blood pressure.

It is important to note that not all people with diabetes will have high blood pressure, and having diabetes does not automatically mean that you will develop hypertension. To lessen the danger of problems, it's crucial to frequently monitor your blood pressure if you have diabetes and to successfully treat both disorders.

Chapter 10

Diabetes and Loss of Weight

Why does diabetes make people lose weight?

There are various ways that diabetes might result in weight loss:

1. Insufficient insulin production: Insulin, a hormone that helps control blood sugar levels, is not produced in sufficient amounts in type 1 diabetes. The body can't adequately use glucose for energy if there isn't enough insulin present.

As a result, the body starts metabolizing fat and muscle for energy, which causes weight loss.

2. Increased urination: Both type 1 and type 2 diabetics with high blood sugar levels might experience excessive thirst and increased urine. This constant urination might cause fluid loss, which then causes weight loss.

3. Inadequate calorie absorption: Type 2 diabetes, in particular, can lead to the body developing insulin resistance, which prevents it from responding to insulin as it should.

Elevated blood sugar levels can result from insulin resistance because the body may find it difficult to transport glucose from the bloodstream into cells.

As a result, the body might not get enough energy from the food it consumes, which could result in weight loss.

4. Calorie loss by urine: In diabetics with extremely high blood sugar levels, the kidneys may attempt to eliminate the extra sugar by excreting it in the urine. As a result, there is an increase in the amount of calories lost as glucose, which results in weight reduction.

5. An elevated metabolic rate: Uncontrolled diabetes, particularly when blood sugar levels are regularly high, can cause this.

The body may burn calories more quickly as a result of this accelerated metabolism, leading to weight loss.

It's crucial to understand that weight loss is not always a sign of diabetes. People with diabetes occasionally gain weight or maintain their weight. Diabetes's impact on weight might vary based on a person's metabolism, general health, course of treatment, and lifestyle choices.

For an accurate diagnosis and suitable management, it's crucial to see a healthcare expert if you're dealing with unexplained weight loss or any other troubling symptoms.